The Keto Diet

There's No Need to Sacrifice Taste

Double Healthy

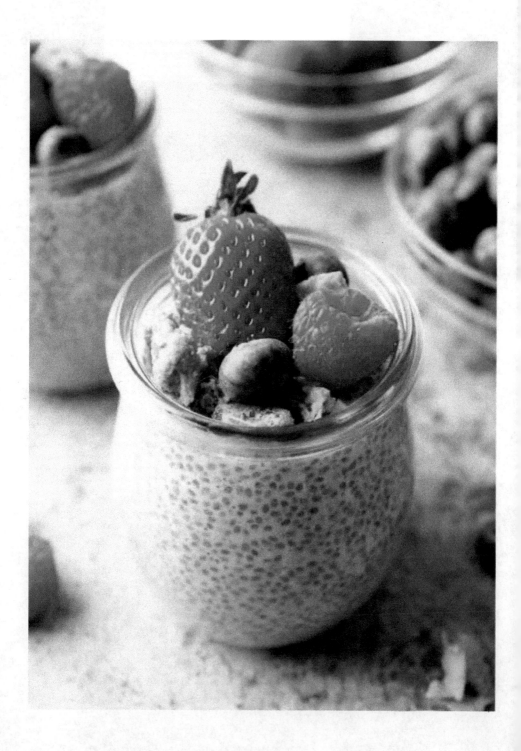

as universal. As befitting its nature, it is presented without assurance regarding its prolonged validity or interim quality. Trademarks that are mentioned are done without written consent and can in no way be considered an endorsement from the trademark holder.

Table of Contents

Introduction

Have you ever looked in the mirror and wondered how to lose weight and get into better shape? How about being free of conditions like high blood pressure and less than ideal cholesterol levels to enjoy a wholesome, healthy, and active life? There is no longer any need to worry about these health issues and others caused by obesity or excess weight. This book will help you live a happier, healthier life.

It provides over 60 easy to follow ketosis diet recipes with complete nutritional information and a one-week healthy and delicious meal plan. Following a ketogenic diet plan has never been this easy before. This book will explain what the keto diet is, what foods are and are not allowed, and lays out a diet plan for a week, along with many easy keto recipes that you can cook at home. Each recipe includes the amount of servings, preparation time, and nutritional information per serving. They will help you feel energized, lose weight, regain your health, and keep you in nutritional ketosis. We have got you covered from morning till night, breakfast to dinner.

The keto diet is an eating plan that is focused on providing a lot of health benefits by knowing how to balance your protein and carbs. Its benefits also involve dissolving or depleting already present fats. Losing weight can be challenging, mainly due to the fact that it involves a certain degree of sacrifice. Unfortunately, there is no good alternative to dieting unless you have painful, risky, and expensive surgeries. But the good news is that you can use the keto diet to lose weight in a healthy and natural way. It is easier than you think to lose those extra pounds, look great, and stay healthy without worrying about negative side-effects.

The ketogenic diet is one of the best and most effective weight loss diets available. Through this keto cookbook, you will learn about how this diet works and how to start your weight loss regimen. This book contains delicious ketogenic recipes for breakfast, lunch, soups, salads, and dinner that are easy to make and perfect for the busy working dieters out there.

If you are just starting out with keto, having a good cookbook designed for beginners can help you adjust to the diet and lose your weight without health issues. The Introduction to Ketogenic Recipes: Ketogenic Diet Cookbook for Beginners is designed to help beginners know the importance of the keto diet, lose weight, and enjoy the ketogenic lifestyle for life.

So Take Advantage of the Benefits From this Awesome Book!

Ketogenic Diets

The ketogenic diet utilizes low carbs and high fat to offer unlimited health benefits. It doesn't only help you in losing weight but also improves your health. It offers benefits against epilepsy, Alzheimer's disease, diabetes, cancer, and obesity. It consists of drastically decreasing carbohydrate intake and replacing it with fat. This creates a metabolic condition called "ketosis," which will cause your body to use fat for fuel instead of carbohydrates. Glucose is the main source of energy for the cells, so when the intake of carbohydrates is reduced, the body's supply of glucose is reduced and causes ketosis.

There has been a lot of talk in nutrition science lately about the huge health advantage of low carb and ketogenic diets. These diets benefit your blood pressure, cholesterol, and blood sugar. They also decrease cravings and appetite, boost weight loss, and lower triglyceride levels. The low-carb and high-fat diet lowers insulin levels and blood sugar and shifts the body's metabolism away from carbs and towards fat and ketones. Adjusting your diet and practicing intermittent fasting can assist you to enter ketosis more quickly. There are home tests that can help in determining when you've entered ketosis.

Foods Included in the Ketogenic Diet:

- Seafood
- Eggs
- Cheese
- Olives
- Coconut oil
- Plain Greek yogurt and cottage cheese
- Low-carb vegetables
- Shirataki Noodles
- Unsweetened Tea
- Butter and Cream
- Avocados
- Meat and poultry
- Dark chocolate and cocoa powder
- Unsweetened coffee
- Nuts and seeds
- Berries

Foods Not Included in the Ketogenic Diet

- Grains
- Starchy vegetables and high-sugar fruits
- Sweetened yogurt
- Juices
- Honey, syrup, or sugar in any form
- Chips and crackers
- Baked goods including gluten-free
- Corn
- Rice
- Potato and sweet potato

Keto Diet Meal Plan

Monday

Breakfast

Sheet pan egg and bacon

Lunch

Broccoli and salad

Dinner

Chicken soup

Tuesday

Breakfast

Keto banana walnut bread and bacon

Lunch

Broccoli and salad

Dinner

Italian steak with cauliflower rice

Wednesday

Breakfast

Sheet pan egg and bacon

Lunch

Loaded chicken salad with veggies

Dinner

Chicken soup

Thursday

Breakfast

Keto banana walnut bread and bacon

Lunch

Loaded chicken salad with veggies

Dinner

Balsamic chicken with broccoli

Friday

Breakfast

Green chili chicken egg cups

Lunch

Cheeseburger soup

Dinner

Chipotle pork with cauliflower rice

Saturday

Breakfast

Cream cheese pancake with bacon

Lunch

Cheeseburger soup

Dinner

Stuffed peppers

Sunday

Breakfast

Sheet egg pan and bacon

Lunch

Keto zucchini pizza bites

Dinner

Red wine beef brisket with asparagus

Drinks and Desserts Recipes

Marshmallows with Chocolate

Servings: 4

Preparation time: 40 minutes

Nutrition per serving: Cal 83; Fat 5.3g; Net Carbs 3.6g; Protein 2.2g

Ingredients:

- 6 tbsp. cool water
- 2 ½ tsp gelatin powder
- ½ cup erythritol
- 1 tbsp. unsweetened cocoa powder

- 2 tbsp. unsweetened cocoa powder
- ½ tsp vanilla extract
- 1 tbsp. xanthan gum mixed in 1 tbsp. water
- A pinch salt
- 1 tbsp. Swerve confectioner's sugar

Procedure:

1. First of all, grease a lined with parchment paper loaf pan with cooking spray and set aside.

2. Then mix the erythritol, 2 tbsp. of water, xanthan gum mixture, and salt in a saucepan.

3. Place the pan over high heat and bring to a boil.

4. After that, insert a thermometer and let the ingredients simmer at 220 F for 8 minutes.

5. Then add 2 tbsp of water and gelatin in a small bowl.

6. Let it sit to dissolve for 5 minutes.

7. While the gelatin dissolves, pour the remaining water into a small bowl and heat in the microwave for 30 seconds.

8. Now stir in cocoa powder and mix it into the gelatin.

9. When the erythritol solution has hit the right temperature, gradually pour it directly into the gelatin mixture, stirring continuously.

10. After that, beat for 12 minutes to get a light and fluffy consistency.

11. Then, stir in the vanilla and pour the blend into the loaf pan.

12. Now let the marshmallows set for 3 hours in the fridge.

13. Use an oiled knife to cut into cubes and place them on a plate.

14. Mix the remaining cocoa powder and confectioner's sugar together.

15. Finally, sift it over the marshmallows.

Citrus Mousse with Almonds

Servings: 8

Preparation time: 15 minutes

Nutrition per serving: Cal 242; Fat 18g; Net Carbs 3.3g; Protein 6.5g

Ingredients:

- 4 cups Swerve confectioner's sugar
- 2 lime, juiced and zested
- Salt to taste
- 2 cup whipped cream + extra for garnish
- 1 lb. cream cheese, softened
- 2 lemon, juiced and zested
- ½ cup toasted almonds, chopped

Procedure:

1. Take a bowl and with a hand mixer, whip the cream cheese until light and fluffy.

2. Then add in the sugar, lemon and lime juices, and salt and mix well.

3. Now fold in the whipped cream to evenly combine.

4. Then spoon the mousse into serving cups and refrigerate to thicken for 1 hour.

5. Swirl with extra whipped cream and garnish with lemon and lime zest.

6. Finally, serve immediately topped with almonds.

Buckeye Bars

Servings: 8

Preparation time: 15 minutes

Nutrition per serving: Cal 409; Net Carbs 5.5g; Fat 38g; Protein 9.8g

Ingredients:

- 1 cup butter, melted
- 2 ½ tps peanut butter
- 2 tsp Swerve sugar
- 12 oz dark chocolate chips
- ¼ tsp salt
- 1 cup almond flour
- 12 oz heavy cream
- 2 tsp vanilla extract

Procedure:

1. Take a food processor, mix butter, almond flour, peanut butter, vanilla, and Swerve sugar.

2. Then line a baking sheet with parchment paper.

3. Spread the vanilla mixture onto the sheet and refrigerate to firm, 30 minutes.

4. After that, add the chocolate chips, heavy cream, and salt to a pot and melt over low heat until bubbles form around the edges.

5. Now let cool for 5 minutes and whisk until smooth.

6. Pour over the butter mixture and refrigerate for 1 hour.

7. Finally, cut into bars and serve.

Berry-Green Smoothie

Servings: 2

Preparation time: 5 minutes

Nutrition per serving: Kcal 360, Fat 33.3g, Net Carbs 6g, Protein 6g

Ingredients:

- 1 ½ cups mixed blueberries and strawberries
- ½ avocado, pitted and sliced
- 1 cups unsweetened almond milk
- 3 tbsp. heavy cream
- 1 tbsp. erythritol
- ½ cup ice cubes
- ¼ cup nuts and seeds mix

Procedure:

1. Firstly, combine the almond milk, avocado slices, nuts, blueberries, heavy cream, erythritol, strawberries, ice cubes, and seeds in a smoothie maker.

2. Then blend at high speed until smooth and uniform.

3. Now pour the smoothie into drinking glasses and serve immediately.

Nut Granola & Smoothie Bowl

Servings: 2

Preparation time: 5 minutes

Nutrition per serving: Kcal 361, Fat 31.2g, Net Carbs 2g, Protein 13g

Ingredients:

- 3 cups Greek yogurt
- 1 ½ tbsp. unsweetened cocoa powder
- 2 tsp swerve brown sugar
- 1 cups nut granola for topping
- 2 tbsp. almond butter
- A handful toasted walnuts

Procedure:

1. Combine the cocoa powder, Greek yogurt, walnuts, almond butter, and swerve brown sugar in a smoothie maker.

2. Then puree at high speed until smooth and well mixed.

3. Share the smoothie into 2 breakfast bowls and top with a half cup of granola each one, and serve.

Almond Shake

Servings: 4

Preparation time: 5 minutes

Nutrition per serving: Kcal 326, Fat: 27g, Net Carbs: 6g, Protein: 19g

Ingredients:

- 3 cups almond milk
- 1 tsp almond extract
- 2 tbsp collagen peptides
- 1 tsp cinnamon
- 30 drops of stevia
- A handful of ice cubes
- 4 tbsp almond butter
- 4 tbsp flax meal
- A pinch of salt

Procedure:

1. First add flax meal, almond extract, almond milk, almond butter, collagen peptides, a pinch of salt, and stevia to a blender bowl.

2. Then blitz until uniform and smooth, about 30 seconds.

3. Then taste and adjust flavor as needed, adding more stevia for sweetness or almond butter to the creaminess.

4. Pour in a smoothie glass and add the ice cubes and sprinkle with cinnamon.

Coconut Protein Shake

Servings: 2

Preparation time: 5 minutes

Nutrition per serving: Kcal 265, Fat: 15.5g, Net Carbs: 4g, Protein: 12g

Ingredients:

- 1 ½ cups flax milk, chilled
- 2 mint leaves + extra to garnish
- 1 ½ tsp unsweetened cocoa powder
- 1 ½ tbsp. erythritol
- ½ tbsp. low carb protein powder
- ½ medium avocado, peeled, sliced
- ½ cup coconut milk, chilled
- Whipping cream for topping

Procedure:

1. Add avocado, coconut milk, mint leaves, erythritol, the flax milk, cocoa powder, and protein powder into the smoothie maker, and blend for 1 minute to smooth.

2. Then pour the drink into serving glasses, lightly add some whipping cream on top.

3. Garnish with 1 or 2 mint leaves. Serve immediately.

Amazing Five Greens Smoothie

Servings: 2

Preparation time: 5 minutes

Nutrition per serving: Kcal 124, Fat 7.8g, Net Carbs 2.9g, Protein 3.2g

Ingredients:

- 1 ½ stalks celery, chopped
- ½ cucumber, peeled and chopped
- Chia seeds to garnish
- ½ ripe avocado, skinned and sliced
- 1 cup spinach, chopped
- kale leaves, chopped

Procedure:

1. Take a blender, add the kale, avocado, ice cubes, and celery and blend for 45 seconds.

2. Then add the spinach and cucumber, and process for another 45 seconds until smooth.

3. After that, pour the smoothie into glasses, garnish with chia seeds, and serve the drink immediately.

Swiss Chard Dip

Servings: 3

Preparation time: 25 minutes

Nutrition per serving: 75 Calories; 3g Fat; 6g Carbs; 2.9g Protein; 0.8g Fiber

Ingredients:

- 1 cup Swiss chard
- ½ teaspoon dried Mediterranean spice mix
- 1 teaspoon sesame oil
- Salt and pepper, to taste
- ¼ cup almond milk
- 1 teaspoon nutritional yeast
- ½ cup tofu, pressed and crumbled
- ½ teaspoon fresh garlic, smashed

Procedure:

1. Firstly, parboil the Swiss chard in a pot of lightly salted water for about 6-7 minutes.
2. Then, transfer the mixture to the bowl of a food processor and add in the other ingredients.
3. After that, process the ingredients until the mixture is homogeneous.
4. Finally, bake in the preheated oven at 390 degrees F for about 10 minutes.

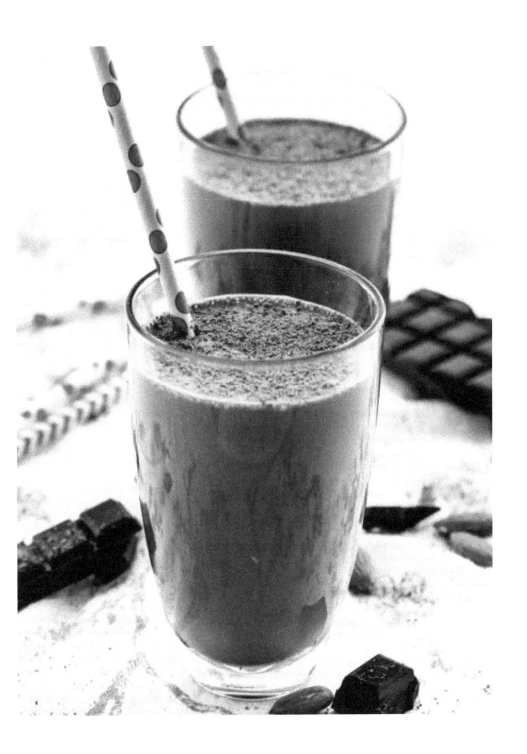

Chocolate Smoothie

Servings: 4

Preparation time: 10 minutes

Nutrition per serving: 335 Calories; 31.7g Fat; 5.7g Carbs; 7g Protein; 1.9g Fiber

Ingredients:

1. 2 tablespoon chia seeds
2. 1 cup coconut milk
3. 1 cup water
4. 3 cups baby spinach
5. 2 tablespoon unsweetened cocoa powder
6. 4 tablespoons Swerve
7. 16 almonds

Procedure:

1. Take a blender, add all the ingredients.
2. Blend well for 45-50 minutes.
3. Serve.

Oats with Mixed Berries

Servings: 2

Preparation time: 5 minutes

Nutrition per serving: 176 Calories; 12.7g Fat; 6g Carbs; 9.7g Protein; 3.2g Fiber

Ingredients:

1. ¼ teaspoon ground cinnamon
2. ¼ cup hemp hearts
3. 3 tbsp. sunflower seeds
4. ¼ cup coconut milk, unsweetened
5. ½ cup mixed berries
6. 4 tablespoons granulated Swerve
7. ¼ cup water

Procedure:

1. Firstly, combine the water, sunflower seeds, Swerve, milk, hemp hearts, and cinnamon in an airtight container.
2. Cover and let it stand in your refrigerator overnight.

Chia Pudding

Servings: 6

Preparation time: 5 minutes

Nutrition per serving: 153 Calories; 8g Fat; 6.7g Carbs; 6.7g Protein; 2.6g Fiber

Ingredients:

- 18 blackberries, fresh or frozen
- ½ teaspoon ground cloves
- ½ teaspoon grated nutmeg
- ½ cup hemp hearts
- 4 cups coconut milk, unsweetened
- ½ cup chia seeds
- ¼ teaspoon coarse sea salt
- A few drops of liquid Stevia
- ½ teaspoon ground cinnamon

Procedure:

1. First combine the chia seeds, salt, ground cloves, coconut milk, hemp hearts, nutmeg, cinnamon, and Stevia in an airtight container.
2. Cover and let it stand in your refrigerator overnight.

Simple Keto Recipes

Greenish Cheesy Bowls

Servings: 2

Preparation time: 10 minutes

Nutrition per serving: Cal 323; Net Carbs 8.1g; Fat 26g; Protein 15g

Ingredients:

- ¼ cup baby kale
- ¼ cup crumbled feta cheese
- ½ tbsp. dill, chopped
- 1 tbsp. toasted pine nuts
- Salt and black pepper to taste
- 1 zucchinis, spiralized
- ¼ cup crumbled goat cheese
- ¼ lemon, juiced
- ½ tbsp. olive oil

Procedure:

1. Firstly, place the zucchinis in a bowl and season with salt and pepper.

2. Take a small bowl, mix the olive oil, lemon juice, and mustard.

3. Then, pour the mixture over the zucchini and toss evenly.

4. Add the dill, kale, goat cheese, feta cheese, and pine nuts. Toss to combine and serve.

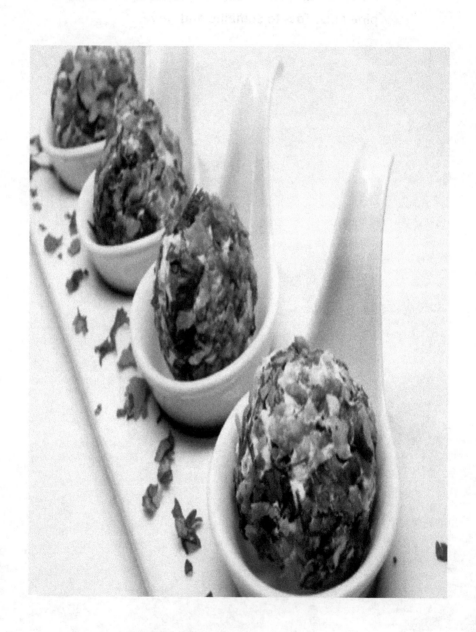

Bacon Fat Bombs with Cheese

Servings: 6

Preparation time: 45 minutes

Nutrition per serving: Cal 282; Net Carbs 0.1g; Fat 26g; Protein 11g

Ingredients:

- 4 tbsp. butter, softened
- 8 bacon slices, chopped
- ½ cup Chevre cheese, grated
- ½ cup cream cheese, softened

Procedure:

1. Firstly, fry the bacon in a skillet over medium heat for 5 minutes.

2. Then grease a baking sheet with the bacon fat and set aside.

3. Take a bowl, stir together the cream cheese, Chèvre cheese, butter, and stir-fried bacon until well blended.

4. Roll the mixture into 12 "balls" and place them on the sheet.

5. Finally freeze for 30 minutes.

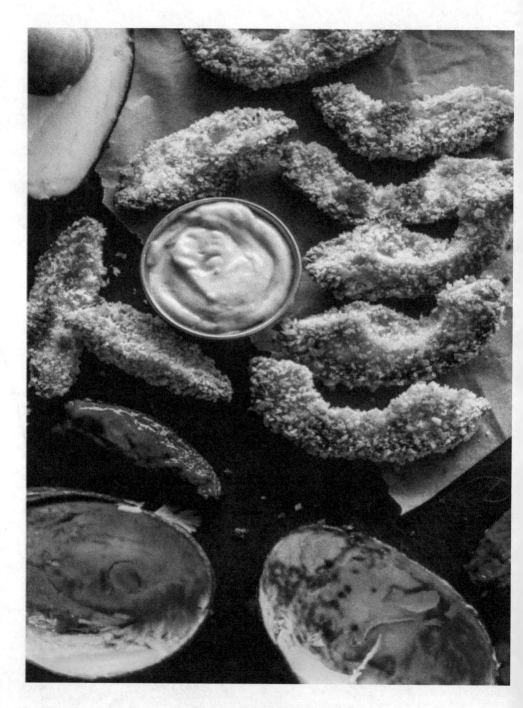

Avocado Fries with Sauce

Servings: 2

Preparation time: 20 minutes

Nutrition per serving: Cal 633; Net Carbs 2.7g; Fat 58g; Protein 11g

Ingredients:

- 1 tbsp. lemon juice
- 1 avocados, sliced
- ½ cup almond flour
- 1 chipotle sauce
- ¼ cup mayonnaise
- Salt and black pepper to taste
- 3 tbsp. olive oil
- 1 large egg, beaten

Procedure:

1. First mix the almond flour with salt and black pepper.

2. Then toss avocado slices in the eggs and then dredge in the flour mixture.

3. Now heat olive oil in a deep pan and fry the avocado slices until golden brown, 2-3 minutes per side.

4. Take a bowl, mix the lemon juice, chipotle sauce, mayonnaise, and salt.

5. Serve the fries with the sauce.

Pigs in Blanket

Servings: 2

Preparation time: 30minutes

Nutrition per serving: Cal 620; Net Carbs 0g; Fat 56g; Protein 28g

Ingredients:

- 4 Vienna sausages
- 4 thin bacon slices

Procedure:

1. Preheat oven to 360 F.

2. Wrap each sausage tightly with a slice of bacon.

3. Lay the bacon-wrapped sausages on a greased baking sheet and roast for 18-20 minutes until the bacon is crisp and golden.

4. Top with rosemary.

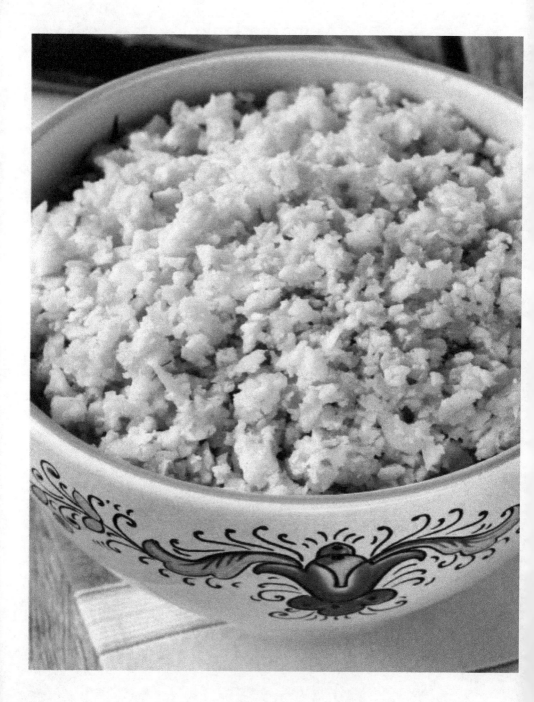

Saffron Cauliflower Rice

Servings: 2

Preparation time: 15 minutes

Nutrition per serving: Cal 89; Net Carbs 5.9g; Fat 6g;
Protein 2g

Ingredients:

- ½ tbsp. butter
- ½ yellow onion, thinly sliced
- 1 cups cauliflower rice
- 3 tbsp. vegetable broth
- 1 tbsp. olive oil
- 3 garlic cloves, sliced
- 1 tbsp. chopped parsley
- Salt and black pepper to taste

- A pinch of saffron soaked in ¼-cup almond milk

Procedure:

1. First warm olive oil in a saucepan over medium
   heat and fry garlic until golden brown but not
   burned; set aside.

2. Then, sauté butter and onion in a saucepan for 3
   minutes.

3. After that, stir in cauliflower rice.

4. Now remove the saffron from the milk and pour the milk and stock into the saucepan.

5. Mix, cover, and cook for 5 minutes.

6. Season it with salt, black pepper, and parsley.

7. Now fluff the cauli rice and dish into serving plates.

8. Finally, garnish with the fried garlic and serve.

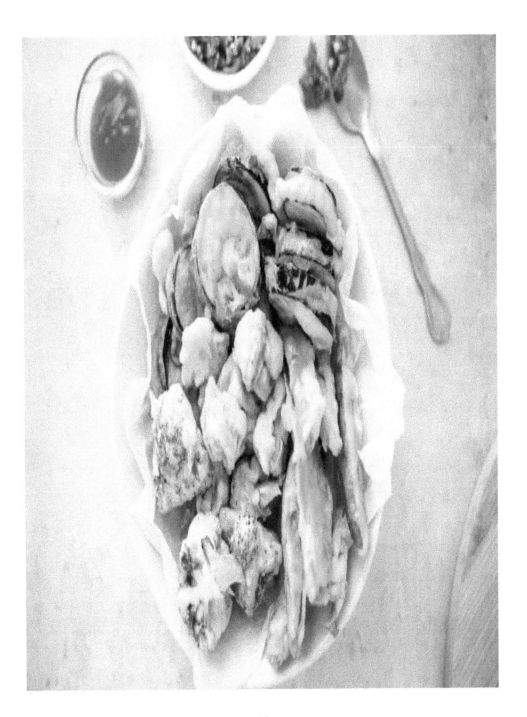

Vegetable Tempura

Servings: 2

Preparation time: 20 minutes

Nutrition per serving: Kcal 218, Fat 17g, Net Carbs 0.9g, Protein 3g

Ingredients:

- ¼ cup coconut flour + extra for dredging
- ½ cup chilled water
- 2 lemon wedge
- ¼ cup sugar-free soy sauce
- Salt and black pepper to taste
- 2 egg yolks
- 1 red bell pepper, cut into strips
- 2 tbsp olive oil
- ½ squash, peeled and cut into strips
- ½ broccoli, cut into florets

Procedure:

1. Take a deep frying pan, heat the olive oil over medium heat.

2. Then beat the eggs lightly with ½ cup of coconut flour and water.

3. The mixture should be lumpy.

4. Now dredge the vegetables lightly in some flour, shake off the excess flour, dip it in the batter, and then into the hot oil.

5. Then fry in batches for 1 minute each, not more, and remove with a perforated spoon onto a wire rack.

6. Finally sprinkle with salt and pepper and serve with the lemon wedges and soy sauce.

Green Bean Crisps

Servings: 6

Preparation time: 30 minutes

Nutrition per serving: Kcal 210, Fat 19g, Net Carbs 3g, Protein 5g

Ingredients:

- ¼ cup Pecorino cheese, grated
- 2 eggs
- 1 lb green beans, thread removed
- 1 tsp garlic powder
- Salt and black pepper to taste
- ¼ cup pork rind crumbs

Procedure:

1. First preheat oven to 425ºF and line a baking sheet with foil.

2. Then mix the cheese, garlic powder, salt, pork rinds, and black pepper in a bowl.

3. Beat the eggs in another bowl.

4. Now coat green beans in eggs, then cheese mixture, and arrange evenly on the baking sheet.

5. After that grease lightly with cooking spray and bake for 15 minutes to be crispy.

6. Transfer to a wire rack to cool before serving.

7. In conclusion serve with sugar-free tomato dip.

Prosciutto Wraps

Servings: 3

Preparation time: 15 minutes

Nutrition per serving: Kcal 163, Fat: 12g, Net Carbs: 0.1g, Protein: 13g

Ingredients:

- 1 tbsp. extra virgin olive oil
- 3 thin prosciutto slices
- 9 basil leaves
- 9 ciliegine mozzarella balls

Procedure:

1. First cut the prosciutto slices into three strips each.

2. Then place basil leaves at the end of each strip.

3. After that, top with a ciliegine mozzarella ball.

4. Wrap the mozzarella in prosciutto.

5. Now secure with toothpicks.

6. Arrange on a platter, drizzle with olive oil, and serve.

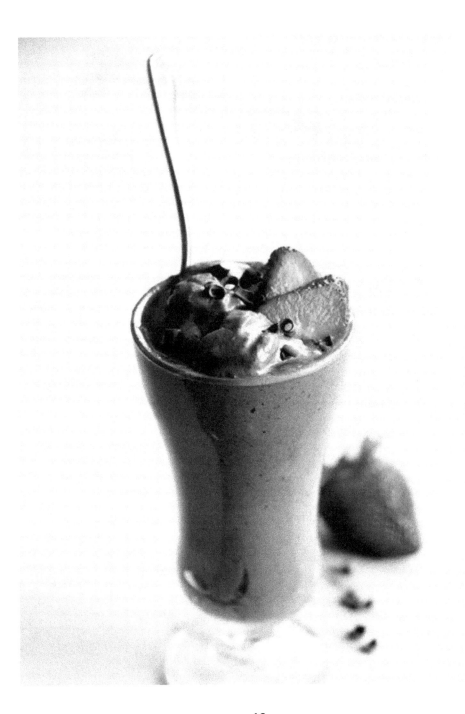

Berry Chocolate Shake

Servings: 4

Preparation time: 10 minutes

Nutrition per serving: 103 Calories; 5.9g Fat; 6.1g Carbs; 4.1g Protein; 2.4g Fiber

Ingredients:

- 2 cup mixed berries
- 2 tablespoon flax seeds, ground
- 2 tablespoon cocoa, unsweetened
- 1 teaspoon ground cinnamon
- 4 tablespoons Swerve
- 2 cup water
- 2 tablespoon peanut butter
- ½ teaspoon ground cloves

Procedure:

1. Add all ingredients in a blender and blend until smooth, creamy, and uniform.

Celery and Carrot Salad

Servings: 6

Preparation time: 10 minutes

Nutrition per serving: 196 Calories; 17.2g Fat; 6g Carbs; 1.2g Protein; 2.2g Fiber

Ingredients:

- ½ pound carrots, coarsely shredded
- ½ cup fresh parsley, chopped
- 1 ¼ pound celery, shredded
- 2 lemon, freshly squeezed
- 4 tablespoons balsamic vinegar
- 1 teaspoon ground allspice
- 1 teaspoon Sriracha sauce
- For the Vinaigrette:
- 4 garlic cloves, smashed
- Sea salt and pepper, to taste
- ¼ cup olive oil

Procedure:

1. First toss the celery, carrots, and parsley in a bowl until everything is well combined.
2. Then mix all ingredients for vinaigrette and dress your salad.

Pine Nuts and Cubed Tofu

Servings: 2

Preparation time: 12 minutes

Nutrition per serving: 232 Calories; 21.6g Fat; 5.3g Carbs; 8.3g Protein; 2.4g Fiber

Ingredients:

- ½ cup extra firm tofu, pressed and cubed
- 1 ½ teaspoons avocado oil
- 1/3 cup pine nuts, coarsely chopped
- Salt and pepper, to season
- 1 garlic cloves, minced
- ½ teaspoon red pepper flakes
- 1 teaspoons lightly toasted sesame seeds
- ¾ tablespoons coconut aminos
- 1 ½ tablespoons vegetable broth
- ¼ teaspoon porcini powder
- ¼ teaspoon ground cumin

Procedure:

1. Take a wok, heat the avocado oil over a moderately-high heat.
2. Now, fry the tofu cubes for 5 to 6 minutes until golden brown on all sides.

3. Then stir in the broth, garlic, red pepper, pecans, coconut aminos, porcini powder, cumin, salt, and pepper and continue to stir for about 8 minutes.
4. Finally top with toasted sesame seeds.

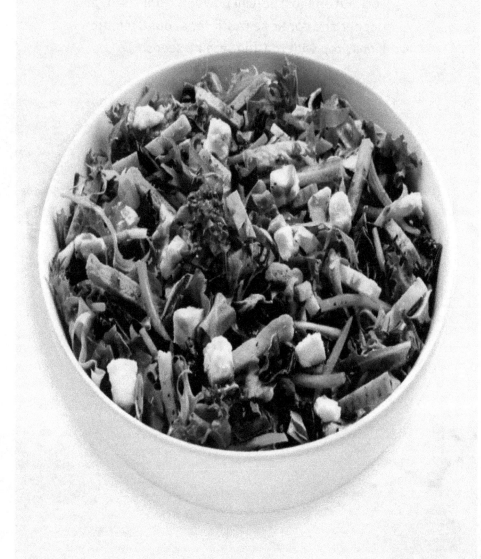

Mediterranean Crunchy Salad

Servings: 8

Preparation time: 15mminutes

Nutrition per serving: 208 Calories; 15.6g Fat; 6.2g Carbs; 7.6g Protein; 6g Fiber

Ingredients:

- 4 tablespoons onions, chopped
- 1 cup almond milk
- 1 teaspoon garlic, chopped
- 1 teaspoon paprika
- 4 tablespoons black olives, pitted
- 2 cup sunflower seeds, soaked overnight
- 2 lemon, freshly squeezed
- 2 Lebanese cucumbers, sliced
- 2 head Romaine lettuce, separated into leaves
- 2 tablespoon cilantro leaves, coarsely chopped
- 1 teaspoon Mediterranean herb mix
- Salt and pepper, to taste
- 2 cup cherry tomatoes, halved

Procedure:

- Fits process all of the dressing ingredients until creamy and smooth.

- Then toss all of the salad ingredients in a bowl. Dress your salad.

Keto Poultry Recipes

Chicken Stew

Preparation time: 1 hour

Nutrition per serving: 280 Calories; 14.7g Fat; 2.5g Carbs; 25.6g Protein; 2.5g Fiber

Ingredients:

- ½ pound chicken thighs
- ½ cup tomato puree
- Kosher salt and ground black pepper, to taste
- 1 tablespoons butter, room temperature
- 1/4 pound carrots, chopped
- 1/2 teaspoon garlic, sliced
- 2 cups vegetable broth
- ½ teaspoon dried basil
- ½ celery, chopped
- ½ bell pepper, chopped
- ½ chili pepper, deveined and minced
- 1/4 teaspoon smoked paprika
- ½ onion, finely chopped

Procedure:

1. First melt the butter in a stockpot over medium-high flame.

2. Sweat the onion and garlic until just tender and fragrant.
3. After that, reduce the heat to medium-low.
4. Stir in the broth, chicken thighs, and basil and bring to a rolling boil.
5. Then add in the remaining ingredients.
6. Partially cover and let it simmer for 45 to 50 minutes.
7. Shred the meat, discarding the bones; add the chicken back to the pot.

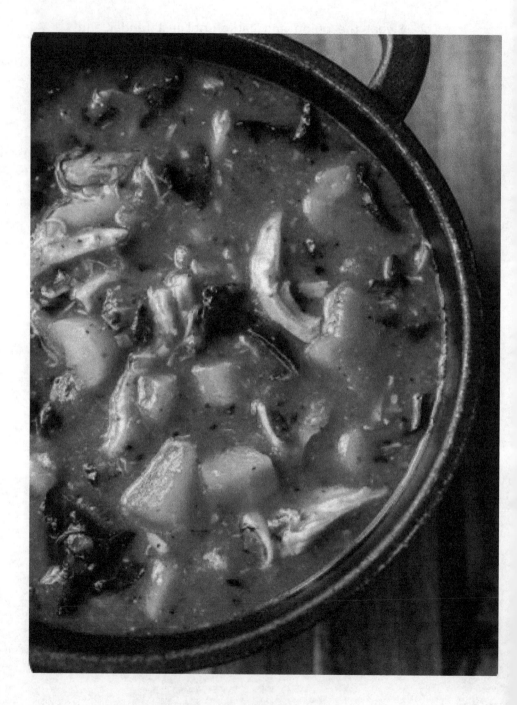

Autumn Chicken Soup

Servings: 2

Preparation time: minutes

Nutrition per serving: 342 Calories; 22.4g Fat; 6.3g Carbs; 25.2g Protein; 1.3g Fiber

Ingredients:

- 1/4 cup turnip, chopped
- 2 cups chicken broth
- ½ tablespoon butter
- ½ teaspoon garlic, finely minced
- ½ cup full-fat milk
- ½ cup double cream
- ¼ parsnip, chopped
- ¼ celery
- 1 small egg
- 1 chicken drumsticks, boneless and cut into small pieces
- Salt and pepper, to taste
- ½ carrot, chopped

Procedure:

1. First melt the butter in a heavy-bottomed pot over medium-high heat and sauté the garlic until aromatic or about 1 minute.

2. Then add in the vegetables and continue to cook until they've softened.
3. Now add in the chicken and cook until it is no longer pink for about 4 minutes.
4. Then season with salt and pepper.
5. After that pour in the chicken broth, milk, and heavy cream and bring it to a boil.
6. Reduce the heat to.
7. Partially cover and continue to simmer for 20 to 25 minutes longer.
8. Finally, fold the beaten egg and stir until it is well incorporated.

Chicken Panna Cotta

Servings: 2

Preparation time: 20 minutes

Nutrition per serving: 306 Calories; 18.3g Fat; 4.7g Carbs; 29.5g Protein; 0g Fiber

Ingredients:

- 1 chicken legs, boneless and skinless
- ½ cup Bleu d' Auvergne, crumbled
- 4 gelatin sheets
- Salt and cayenne pepper, to your liking
- ½ tablespoon avocado oil
- 1 teaspoons granular erythritol
- 1/2 cup double cream
- 1 ½ tablespoons water

Procedure:

1. First of all heat the oil in a frying pan over medium-high heat and fry the chicken for about 10 minutes.
2. Then soak the gelatin sheets in cold water. Cook with the , erythritol, water, creamand Bleu d' Auvergne.
3. Then season with salt and pepper and let it simmer over the low heat, stirring for about 3 minutes. Spoon the mixture into four ramekins.

Special Fried Chorizo Sausage

Servings: 2

Preparation time: 20 minutes

Nutrition per serving: 330 Calories; 17.2g Fat; 4.5g Carbs; 34.4g Protein; 1.6g Fiber

Ingredients:

- 8 ounces smoked turkey chorizo
- ½ cup tomato puree
- 2 scallion stalks, chopped
- 3/4 cup Asiago cheese, grated
- ½ tablespoon dry sherry
- ½ tablespoon extra-virgin olive oil
- 1 tablespoons fresh coriander, roughly chopped
- ½ teaspoon oregano
- ½ teaspoon basil
- ½ teaspoon garlic paste
- Sea salt and ground black pepper, to taste

Procedure:

1. Firstly heat the oil in a frying pan over moderately high heat.
2. Now, brown the turkey chorizo, crumbling with a fork for about 5 minutes.

3. Add in the other ingredients, except for cheese and continue to cook for 10 minutes more or until cooked through.

Chicken Drumsticks in Tomato Sauce

Servings: 4

Preparation time: 1 hour

Nutrition per serving: 488 Calories; 24.5g Fat; 2.1g Carbs; 33.6g Protein; 0.9g Fiber

Ingredients:

- 4 tablespoons sesame oil
- 4 tablespoons balsamic vinegar
- 1 cup marinara sauce
- 2 teaspoon garlic, minced
- Salt and black pepper, to taste
- 2 pound turkey wings
- 2 tablespoon Italian herb mix

Procedure:

1. First place the turkey wings, balsamic vinegar, Italian herb mix, and garlic in a ceramic dish.
2. Then cover and let it marinate for 2 to 3 hours in your refrigerator.
3. Now rub the sesame oil over turkey wings.
4. Grill the turkey wings on the preheated grill for about 1 hour, basting with the reserved marinade.

5. Finally, sprinkle with salt and black pepper to taste.

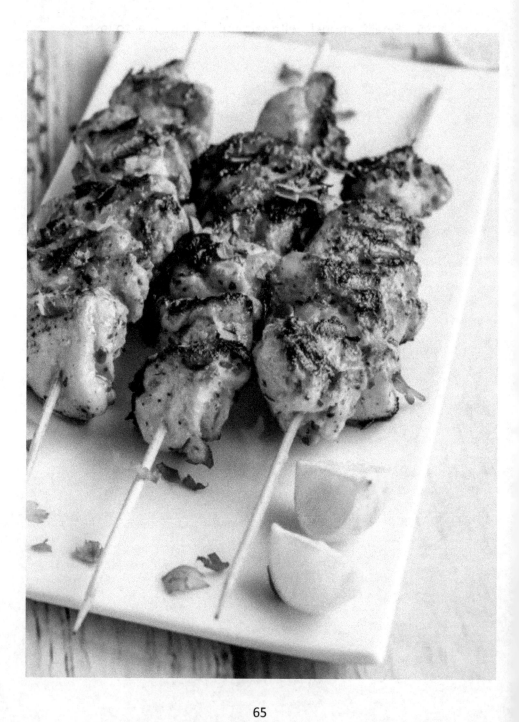

Garlic Chicken Skewers

Servings: 2

Preparation time: 20 minutes

Nutrition per serving: Kcal 225, Fat 17.4g, Net Carbs 2g, Protein 15g

Ingredients:

- 1 1/2 tbsp soy sauce
- 1 tbsp olive oil
- ½ tbsp ginger-garlic paste
- 1 tbsp swerve brown sugar
- ¼ tsp garlic powder
- Pink salt to taste
- ½ tsp chili pepper
- 1/2 lb chicken breasts, cut into cube
- ¼ cup tahini

Procedure:

1. Take a bowl, whisk soy sauce, ginger-garlic paste, swerve brown sugar, chili pepper, and olive oil.

2. Then put the chicken in a zipper bag. Pour in the marinade, seal, and shake to coat. Marinate in the fridge for 2 hours.

3. Meanwhile, preheat grill to 400ºF.

4. Then thread the chicken on skewers. Cook for 10 minutes in total with three to four turnings until golden brown; remove to a plate.

5. Mix the tahini, garlic powder, salt, and ¼ cup of warm water in a bowl.

6. Now pour into serving jars.

7. Finally serve the chicken skewers and tahini dressing with cauli rice.

Chicken in White Wine Sauce

Servings: 4

Preparation time: 40 minutes

Nutrition per serving: Kcal 345, Fat 12g, Net Carbs 4g, Protein 24g

Ingredients:

- 1 ½ chicken thighs
- 4 pancetta strips, chopped
- 10 oz white mushrooms, halved
- 1 cup white wine
- 1 cup whipping cream
- Salt and black pepper to taste
- 2 shallots, chopped
- 2 tbsp canola oil
- 2 garlic cloves, minced

Procedure:

1. First warm the canola oil a pan over medium heat.

2. Then cook the pancetta for 3 minutes.

3. Add in the chicken, sprinkle with pepper and salt, and cook until brown, about 5 minutes.

4. Remove to a plate.

5. Take the same pan, sauté shallots, mushrooms, and garlic for 6 minutes.

6. Return the pancetta and chicken to the pan.

7. Stir in the white wine and 1 cup of water and bring to a boil.

8. Reduce the heat and simmer for 20 minutes.

9. Finally, pour in the whipping cream and warm without boiling. Serve with steamed asparagus.

Yogurt Sauce & Parmesan Wings

Servings: 3

Preparation time: 25 minutes

Nutrition per serving: Kcal 452, Fat 36.4g, Net Carbs 4g, Protein 24g

Ingredients:

- ½ cup Greek-style yogurt
- ¼ cup butter, melted
- ¼ cup hot sauce
- 3 tbsp. Parmesan cheese, grated
- 1 lb chicken wings
- 1 tbsp extra-virgin olive oil
- ½ tbsp fresh dill, chopped
- Salt and black pepper to taste

Procedure:

1. Firstly, preheat oven to 400ºF.
2. After that mix yogurt, olive oil, dill, salt, and black pepper in a bowl.
3. Now chill while making the chicken.
4. Season wings with salt and pepper.
5. After that line them on a baking sheet and grease with cooking spray.

6. Now bake for 20 minutes until golden brown.

7. Mix butter, hot sauce, and Parmesan cheese in a bowl.

8. Then toss chicken in the sauce to evenly coat and plate.

9. Finally serve with yogurt dipping sauce.

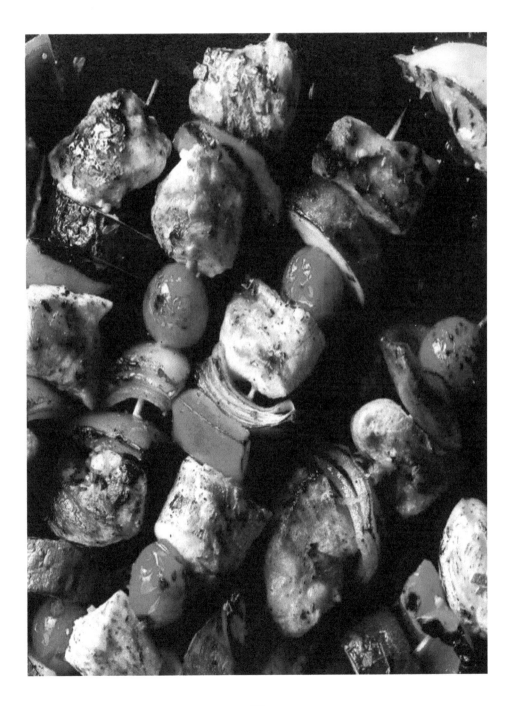

Chicken Lemon Skewers

Servings: 4

Preparation time: 20 minutes

Nutrition per serving: Kcal 350, Fat 11g, Net Carbs 3.5g, Protein 34g

Ingredients:

- 1 lb chicken breasts, cut into cubes
- 2 garlic cloves, minced
- 2 tbsp olive oil
- Salt and black pepper to taste
- 1 tsp fresh rosemary, chopped
- 4 lemon wedges
- 2/3 jar preserved lemon, drained
- ½ cup lemon juice

Procedure:

1. Take wide bowl, mix half of the oil, salt, pepper, garlic, and lemon juice and add the chicken cubes and lemon rind.

2. Then let marinate for 2 hours in the refrigerator.

3. Remove the chicken and thread it onto skewers.

4. Now heat a grill pan over high heat.

5. After that, add in the chicken skewers and sear them for 6 minutes per side.

6. Finally remove to a plate and serve warm garnished with rosemary and lemons wedges.

Fried Chicken with Anchovy Tapenade

Servings: 4

Preparation time: 20 minutes

Nutrition per serving: Cal 522; Fat 37g; Net Carbs 5.3g; Protein 43g

Ingredients:

- ½ cup fresh basil, chopped
- 2 tbsp lemon juice
- 4 tbsp. olive oil
- 2 cup black olives, pitted
- 2 oz anchovy fillets, rinsed
- 2 chicken breasts, cut into 4 pieces
- 4 tbsp. olive oil
- 2 garlic cloves, minced
- 2 garlic clove, crushed
- Salt and black pepper to taste

Procedure:

1. First heat a pan over medium heat and add olive oil.

2. Stir in the garlic and cook for 2 minutes.

3. Then place in the chicken pieces and cook each side for 4 minutes.

4. Now remove to a serving plate.

5. Then chop the black olives and anchovy and put them in a food processor.

6. Add in basil, lemon juice, olive oil, salt, and black pepper, and blend well.

7. Then spoon the tapenade over the chicken and serve.

Chicken Gumbo

Servings: 2

Preparation time: 40 minutes

Nutrition per serving: Cal 433; Fat 26g; Net Carbs 8.7g; Protein 36g

Ingredients:

- ½ stick celery, chopped
- ½ onion, chopped
- ½ cup tomatoes, chopped
- 1 tbsp. cajun seasoning
- 1 ½ tbsp. olive oil

- ½ sausage, sliced
- 1 chicken breast, cubed
- ½ tbsp. sage, chopped
- 2 cups chicken broth
- 1 tbsp. garlic powder
- ½ bay leaf
- ½ bell pepper, chopped
- 1 tbsp. dry mustard
- ½ tbsp. chili powder
- Salt and black pepper, to taste

Procedure:

1. First, heat olive oil in a saucepan over medium heat.

2. Then add the sausage and chicken and cook for 5 minutes.

3. Now add the remaining ingredients, except for the sage, and bring to a boil.

4. Then simmer for 25 minutes.

5. Finally serve sprinkled with sage.

Salami & Cheddar Chicken

Servings: 2

Preparation time: 40 minutes

Nutrition per serving: Cal 417; Fat 25g; Net Carbs 5.2g; Protein 29g

Ingredients:

- ½ tbsp olive oil
- ¾ cups canned tomato sauce
- 2 oz cheddar cheese, sliced
- ½ tsp garlic powder
- Salt and black pepper, to taste
- 1 oz salami, sliced
- ½ lb chicken breasts, halved
- ½ tsp dried oregano

Procedure:

1. First preheat oven to 380 F.

2. Take a bowl, combine oregano, garlic, salt, and pepper.

3. Then rub the chicken with the mixture.

4. Now eat a pan with the olive oil over medium heat, add in the chicken and cook each side for 2 minutes.

5. Remove to a baking dish.

6. After that, top with the cheddar cheese, pour the tomato sauce over, and arrange the salami slices on top.

7. Bake for 30 minutes and serve warm.

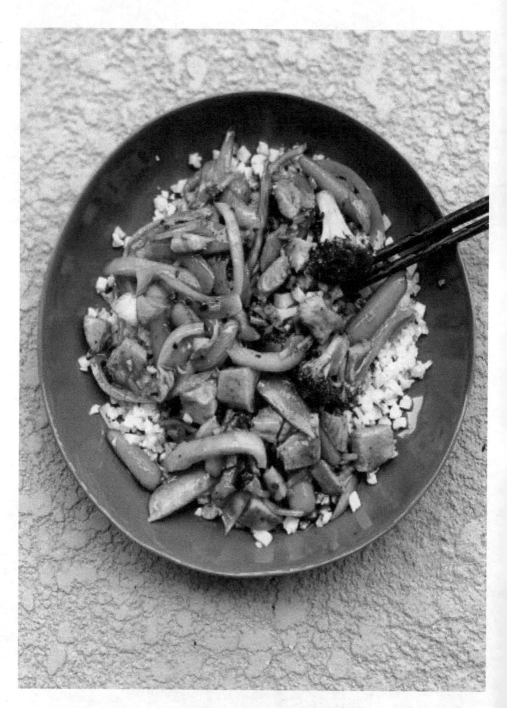

81

Chicken Stir-Fry with Cauliflower

Servings: 2

Preparation time: 25 minutes

Nutrition per serving: Cal 339; Net Carbs 3.5g; Fat 21g; Protein 32g

Ingredients:

- 1 chicken breast, sliced
- 1 ½ tbsp. chicken broth
- 1 tbsp. chopped parsley
- ½ large head cauliflower, cut into florets
- 1 tbsp. olive oil
- ½ red bell pepper, diced
- ½ yellow bell pepper, diced

Procedure:

1. First warm olive oil in a skillet and brown the chicken until brown on all sides, 8 minutes.
2. Then transfer to a plate.
3. Now pour bell peppers into the pan and sauté until softened, 5 minutes.
4. After that, add in cauliflower and broth and stir.
5. Cover the pan and cook for 5 minutes or until cauliflower is tender.
6. Finally mix in chicken and parsley and serve immediately.

Keto Favorite Recipes

Rich Chia Pudding

Servings: 8

Preparation time: 35 minutes

Nutrition per serving: 93 Calories; 5.1g Fat; 7.2g Carbs; 4.4g Protein; 0.7g Fiber

Ingredients:

- 1 ½ cup coconut milk, preferably homemade
- 4 tablespoons peanut butter
- 6 tablespoons orange flower water
- 1 cup chia seeds
- 2 teaspoon liquid Monk fruit
- ½ cup water
- 4 tablespoons chocolate chunks, unsweetened

Procedure:
1. First, thoroughly combine the coconut milk, chia seeds, Monk fruit, water, peanut butter, and orange flower water.
2. Then let the mixture stand for 30 minutes in your refrigerator.
3. Scatter the chopped chocolate over the top of each serving.

Mezze Platter

Servings: 2

Preparation time: 20 minutes

Nutrition per serving: 542 Calories; 46.4g Fat; 6.2g Carbs; 23.7g Protein; 4g Fiber

Ingredients:

- 6 ounces Halloumi cheese, cut into 1/4-1/3-inch slices
- 1 1/2 teaspoons olive oil
- 1/2 teaspoon Greek seasoning blend
- 1/2 tablespoon olive oil
- 3 eggs
- Sea salt and ground black pepper, to taste
- 1/3 cups avocado, pitted and sliced
- ½ cup grape tomatoes, halved
- 2 tablespoons Kalamata olives

Procedure:

1. First preheat a grill pan over medium-high heat, about 400 degrees F.
2. Then grill your halloumi for about 3 minutes or until golden brown grill marks appear.
3. Now heat the oil in a nonstick skillet over moderately-high plate and scramble the eggs with a wide spatula.

Mascarpone Fat Bombs with Bacon

Servings: 2

Preparation time: 15 minutes

Nutrition per serving: 88 Calories; 6.5g Fat; 0.7g Carbs; 6.5g Protein; 0.3g Fiber

Ingredients:

- 2 bacon slices, chopped
- 1/2 teaspoon paprika
- 1/2 teaspoon onion powder
- 1/4 teaspoon garlic powder
- 1/4 cup mascarpone cheese
- 1/4 teaspoon smoke flavor

Procedure:

1. First thoroughly combine all ingredients until well combined.
2. Then roll the mixture into bite-sized balls.

Tortilla Pizza from Spain

Servings: 4

Preparation time: 15 minutes

Nutrition per serving: 397 Calories; 31g Fat; 6.1g Carbs; 22g Protein; 1.4g Fiber

Ingredients:

- 8 eggs, beaten
- 1 teaspoon coriander, minced
- 4 tablespoons flax seed meal
- 2 teaspoon chili pepper, deveined and minced
- 4 ounces Manchego cheese, shredded
- 2 tablespoon extra-virgin olive oil
- 4 tablespoons tomato paste
- Salt and pepper, to taste
- 1/2 cup cream cheese

Procedure:

1. First take a mixing bowl, combine ingredients for the crust.
2. Then divide the batter into two pieces.
3. Now cook in a frying pan for about 5 minutes and flip your tortilla and cook on the other side until crisp and golden-brown on their edges.
4. Then repeat with another tortilla.

5. Spread the tomato paste and cheese over the top of each of the prepared tortillas.
6. In the end place under the preheated broiler for about 5 minutes until the cheese is hot and bubbly.

Stuffed Avocado with Tomato & Cheese

Servings: 8

Preparation time: 25 minutes

Nutrition per serving: 264 Calories; 24.4g Fat; 6g Carbs; 3.7g Protein; 5g Fiber

Ingredients:

- 4 avocados, halved and pitted
- 2 teaspoon olive oil
- 16 black olives, pitted and sliced
- 1 cup tomatoes, chopped
- 6 ounces mascarpone cheese

Procedure:

1. Preheat the oven at 365 degrees

2. Then mix the olive oil, tomatoes, cheese and black olives in a bowl.

3. Spoon the mixture into the avocado halves.
4. Bake in the preheated for about 20 minutes or until everything is cooked through.

Tofu & Avocado Sandwiches

Servings: 4

Preparation time: 10 minutes

Nutrition per serving: Cal 390; Net Carbs 4g; Fat 29g; Protein 12g

Ingredients:

- 8 little gem lettuce leaves
- 1 oz butter, softened
- 2 avocado, sliced
- 2 tsp chopped parsley
- 8 tofu slices
- 2 large red tomato, sliced

Procedure:

1. First place the lettuce on a flat serving plate.

2. Then smear each leaf with butter and arrange tofu slices on the leaves.

3. Now top with the avocado and tomato slices.

4. Finally garnish the sandwiches with parsley and serve.

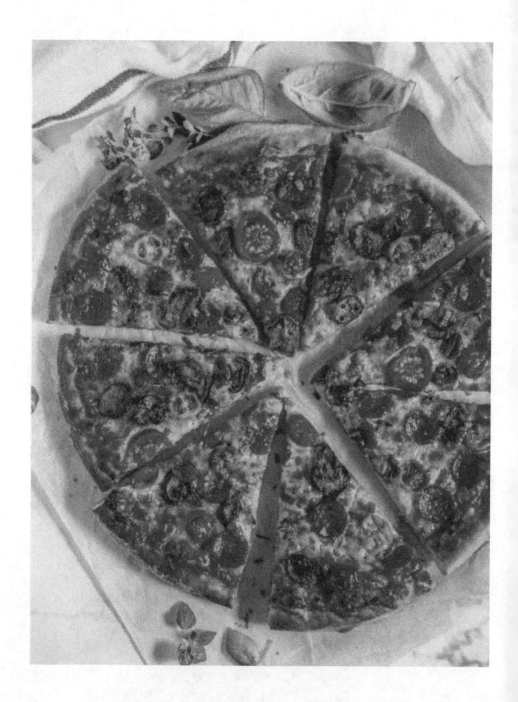

Pepperoni & Mushroom Pizza

Servings: 4

Preparation time: 25 minutes

Nutrition per serving: Cal 512; Fat 41g; Net Carbs 4.6g; Protein 28g

Ingredients:

- 4 (2 pack) cauliflower pizza crusts
- Salt and black pepper to taste
- 1 ½ cup mozzarella, shredded
- 4 oz. mixed mushrooms, sliced
- 2 tbsp. basil pesto
- 4 tbsp. olive oil
- 8 oz. pepperoni, sliced

Procedure:

1. Firstly, preheat the oven to 350 F.

2. Grease two baking dishes with cooking spray.

3. Then add in the two cauliflower crusts.

4. Take a bowl, mix the mushrooms with pesto, olive oil, salt, and black pepper.

5. Now divide the mozzarella cheese on top of the pizza crusts.

6. After that, spread the mushroom mixture and cover with the pepperoni slices.

7. Bake the pizzas in batches until the cheese has melted, about 8 minutes.

8. Finally, remove when ready, cut, and serve with a spinach salad.

Special Gorgonzola & Ricotta Stuffed Peppers

Servings: 2

Preparation time: 55 minutes

Nutrition per serving: Cal 541; Fat 43g; Net Carbs 7.3g; Protein 25g

Ingredients:

- 1/2 cup ricotta cheese
- ¼ cup gorgonzola cheese, crumbled
- ½ tsp dried basil
- Salt and black pepper to taste
- ¼ tsp oregano
- 1 tbsp. olive oil
- 2 red bell peppers, halved
- 1 cloves garlic, minced
- ¾ cups tomatoes, chopped

Procedure:

1. First preheat oven to 360 F and lightly grease the sides and bottom of a baking dish with cooking spray.

2. Take a bowl, mix garlic, tomatoes, gorgonzola and ricotta cheeses.

3. After that, stuff the pepper halves and place them on the baking dish.

4. Now season it with salt, black pepper, oregano, and basil.

5. Finally drizzle with olive oil and bake for 40 minutes until the peppers are tender.

Raw Coconut Balls

Servings: 2

Preparation time: 55 minutes

Nutrition per serving: Cal 541; Fat 43g; Net Carbs 7.3g; Protein 25g

Ingredients:

- 1/4 cup gorgonzola cheese, crumbled
- 1/2 tsp dried basil
- Salt and black pepper to taste
- 1/2 cup ricotta cheese
- 1 cloves garlic, minced
- 1/4 tsp oregano
- 1 tbsp olive oil
- 2 red bell peppers, halved
- 3/4 cups tomatoes, chop

Procedure:

1. First preheat oven to 360 F and lightly grease the sides and bottom of a baking dish with cooking spray.
2. Take a bowl, mix garlic, tomatoes, gorgonzola and ricotta cheeses.

3. Then stuff the pepper halves and place them on the baking dish.

4. After that, season it with salt, black pepper, oregano, and basil.

5. Then drizzle with olive oil and bake for 40 minutes until the peppers are tender.

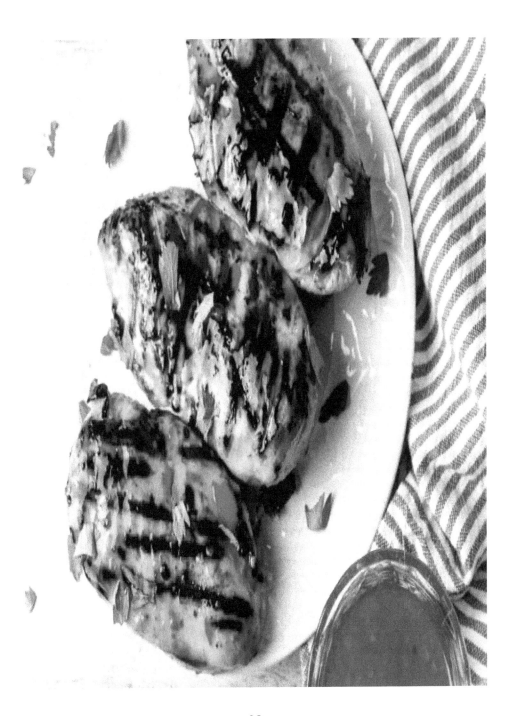

Sweet Chili Grilled Chicken

Servings: 3

Preparation time: 30 minutes

Nutrition per serving: Kcal 265, Fat 9g, Net Carbs 3g, Protein 26g

Ingredients:

- 1 lb. chicken breasts
- Salt and black pepper to taste
- 1 1/2 small chilies, minced
- 2 cloves garlic, minced
- 1/4 cup lemon juice
- ¼ cup olive oil
- 1/2 tbsp. erythritol
- 1 tbsp. fresh oregano, chopped

Procedure:

1. First preheat grill to high heat.

2. Take a bowl, mix the garlic, olive oil, chilies, erythritol, oregano, and lemon juice.

3. Then cover the chicken with plastic wraps and use the rolling pin to pound to ½-inch thickness.

4. Remove the wrap and brush the spice mixture on the chicken on all sides.

5. Now place on the grill and cook for 15 minutes, flip, and continue cooking for 10 more minutes.

6. Finally, remove to a plate and serve with salad.

Squash & Chicken Traybake

Servings: 2

Preparation time: 50 minutes

Nutrition per serving: Kcal: 411, Fat: 15g, Net Carbs: 5.5g, Protein: 31g

Ingredients:

- ¾ lb chicken thighs
- 1/2 lb butternut squash, cubed
- ¼ cup black olives, pitted
- 3 tbsp. olive oil
- 2 1/2 garlic cloves, sliced
- 2/3 dried oregano

Procedure:

1. First preheat oven to 400ºF.

2. Then place the chicken in a greased baking dish with the skin down.

3. Now place the garlic, olives, and butternut squash around the chicken.

4. After that, drizzle with olive oil.

5. Sprinkle with black pepper, salt, and oregano.

6. Now bin the oven for 45 minutes until golden brown.

7. Serve warm.

Stir-fry chicken with Broccoli

Servings: 2

Preparation time: 30 minutes

Nutrition per serving: Kcal 286, Fat 10.1g, Net Carbs 3.4g, Protein 17.3g

Ingredients:

- 1 chicken breasts, cut into strips
- 1/2 white onion, thinly sliced
- Salt and black pepper to taste
- 1 tbsp olive oil
- ½ cup unsalted cashew nuts
- 1 cups broccoli florets

Procedure:

1. First of all toast the cashew nuts in a dry skillet over medium heat for 2-3 minutes, shaking occasionally.

2. Remove to a plate.

3. Then heat the olive oil in the pan and sauté the onion for 4 minutes until soft and set aside.

4. Now add the chicken to the pan.

5. Cook for 4 minutes.

6. After that, include the broccoli, salt, and black pepper.

7. Stir and cook for 5-6 minutes until tender and add in the onion.

8. Now stir once more, cook for 1 minute, and turn the heat off.

9. Serve the chicken stir-fry topped with the cashew nuts.

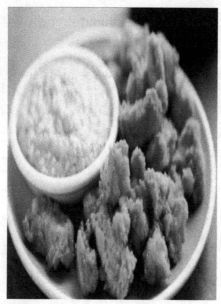

Coconut Sauce and Fried Chicken

Servings: 3

Preparation time: 30 minutes

Nutrition per serving: Kcal 491, Fat 35g, Net Carbs 3.2g, Protein 58g

Ingredients

- 1 1/2 tbsp. coconut oil
- ½ tbsp. lime juice
- 1 lb. chicken breasts
- 1/2 tsp red pepper flakes
- 1 tbsp. green onions, chopped
- Salt and black pepper to taste
- 1/2 cup chicken stock
- ¾ cups leeks, chopped
- 3 tbsp. coconut cream

Procedure:

1. First put a pan over medium heat and warm oil.

2. Secondly, add in the chicken and cook each side for 2 minutes.

3. Set aside.

4. Thirdly, place the leeks in the pan and cook for 4 minutes.

5. Then stir in stock, salt, pepper, coconut cream, pepper flakes, and lime juice.

6. Finally take the chicken back to the pan and cook covered for 15 minutes and serve warm.

CPSIA information can be obtained
at www.ICGtesting.com
Printed in the USA
LVHW080921250321
682295LV00018B/512